Quit Smoking Easily

Quitting Smoking Easily

Quit Smoking Easily

J.Z. Parker

Quitting Smoking Easily

J.Z Parker, Copyright 2024

ISBN: 9798882582288

ALL RIGHTS RESERVED

The author is hereby established as the sole holder of the copyright.

Quitting Smoking Easily

Contents

Quitting Smoking Easily

Quitting Smoking Easily

About the Author

J. Parker believes that each choice you make regarding your food and smoking lifestyle acts as either a deposit into or withdrawal from your "health banking" account. You can choose to make mostly savings deposits or check withdrawals. The balance of that account determines your energy, vitality, risk of disease, longevity, and ultimately the quality of your life.

J. Parker has worked in big food companies creating concepts. J.Z.

is also a pseudonym. J. Parker, fondly referred to as J.P., writes to inspire a healthy relationship with food and exercise, along with practical tips to incorporate healthy living. And yes, he was a bartender at a point in time.

Quitting Smoking Easily

Preface

These days it would be unheard of for people not to smoke. Smoking is a part of everyday life. It was not like this before. Smoking is a fad- although, believe it or not, it has only recently become so.

Most people who smoke cigarettes start the habit as a teenager when they did not know any better.

By the time they realize the damage smoking cigarettes is causing their body system, it is already too late. They are already addicted. Most adults do not pick up smoking cigarettes.

There are more than one thousand million smokers throughout the world. This is an astonishing number, considering the damage smoking does to the body, which we are now all well aware of.

Knowing this, the question "why do people smoke?" is a really complicated one that is being explored much more in depth by many of the world's greatest scientists.

Scientists have shown that smoking causes lung cancer amongst other serious diseases. Scientists have also explained beyond reasonable doubt that passive smoking is also harmful to those that do not smoke.

Whether you smoke 20 cigarettes (one pack) a day or 40 (two packs), there is no doubt that smoking is one killer habit that is extremely bad for you and will seriously affect your health.

It could be one habit you may not live to quit. Cigarettes can make you an offer you cannot refuse because one of those offers is heart attack.

Cigarettes has other offers. It can harm almost every organ in your body. COPD/Emphysema is an avenue of painful slow death. Its crushing and devastating squeeze on your organ is painful to experience. It is like begging for death while you are living a miserable life.

Moreover, it is only now that doctors are beginning to discover the true extent of the harm that smoking can cause to a person's health and to the health of those around him.

Yes, you can. Quit smoking while you are ahead. Smoking over a prolonged period of years can cause you a number of serious diseases and illnesses, some of which are fatal.

The illnesses that will not kill you will leave you with a poorer quality of life in general. You can quit.

Introduction:

Smoking as you well know reduces your life expectancy from approximately 7 years to 30 years. You already know that as a smoker, you are less healthy and less physically fit than your friends who are non-smokers.

You are likely to take more days off from work because you are more likely to suffer illnesses than your non-smoker colleagues. You are also more prone to common illnesses like colds and cough or sore throats.

You are more likely to have infections because your body's immune system is already damaged from smoking.

Smoking cigarettes have long-term negative effects on your health and sometime it is immediate. After you smoke a cigarette your blood pressure will rise and your heart rate will increase.

The heart works and beats faster in the attempt to get your body more oxygen that you just displaced by inhalation of thousands of chemicals one of which is carbon monoxide.

Carbon monoxide, a poisonous gas, will enter the lungs and begin to replace the oxygen. You are slowly killing your heart and your lungs. The tiny hairs in the lungs that filter the air that you breathe will cease to grow and to work because they become paralyzed by the poisonous chemicals that are contained in your cigarette smoke.

Some disease associated with cigarette smoking are:

- Crohn's disease
- Premature aging of the skin
- Loss of smell and taste
- Osteoporosis in women
- Gangrene
- Impotence
- Reduced fertility

There are more deadly disease that you are knowingly inflicting on yourself. They include

- Lung cancer

- Cancer of the mouth
- Cancer of the throat
- Cancer of the larynx
- Cancer of the esophagus
- Stomach cancer
- Kidney cancer
- Cancer of the bladder
- Cancer of the pancreas
- Liver cancer
- Cancer of the penis
- Cancer of the anus
- Cervical cancer
- Prostate cancer

In the long-term, smoking causes other diseases apart from those mentioned above.

- Heart attack
- Coronary heart disease

- Cardiovascular disease
- Congestive heart failure
- Stroke
- Atherosclerosis
- Abdominal aortic aneurysm
- Peripheral artery disease
- Ischemic heart disease
- Angina
- Leukemia

It will be helpful if you as a smoker can imagine if your body can take the punishment of all the above diseases.

Even if your insurance will pay for all the medications, how long can your body take the effects of the various medications that will be prescribed?

And wait, there are more diseases associated with cigarette smoking like:

- Emphysema
- Chronic bronchitis
- Pneumonia

- Asthma
- Diabetes
- Stomach ulcers
- Cataracts
- Gum disease
- High blood pressure

There is no doubt that smoking can have serious consequences for your health, but just how much effect can it have on your life's expectancy? Researchers have concluded that a 30-year-old smoker can expect to live about 36 more years, whereas a 30-year-old non-smoker can expect to live 54 more years.

Scientists have also concluded that the children of a parent or parents who smoke may be at risk from the genetic damage to the parent prior to conception.

There is also the direct effects to the children in the womb, and the passive smoke they are exposed to after they are born.

The amount of life expectancy lost for each pack of cigarettes smoked is 30 minutes, and the years of life expectancy a typical smoker loses is approximately 30 years. A University of California, Berkeley Wellness Letter of April 2000 even has it worse.

The study says that for every cigarette you smoke, it reduces your life by 11 minutes. Thus each carton represents one day and a half of lost life. Every year you smoke a pack a day, you shorten your life by 2 months or 4 months if you are two packs a day smoker

Easiest Ways to Quit Smoking

Smoking is a habit that is insidious and tenacious, and millions of lives are lost every year due to it. It is never too late to stop smoking.

 Addiction can make a smoker rationalize and justify all kinds of crazy notions. Have you read any of my books?

All my books deal with your health. Nothing more. Smoking is an odious, nasty and a killer habit, yet good people still engage in it covering up the odor with colognes and perfumes and mouth washes. Some smokers curse the day they smoked their first cigarette.

For them, it is a day that will live in infamy. They will not tell you that, but yes, they wish they never engaged in smoking.

Not a single intelligent smoker would want any of their off springs to engage in smoking. They know it is a killer habit they purchase with their hard earned money. It is a double whammy.

You may be wondering which smoking-related disease is the number one cause of death among smokers.

If you are thinking it is lung cancer or COPD/Emphysema, you are wrong. While both of these smoking-related diseases do claim a lot of lives, it is heart disease that holds the top slot in the list of diseases that kill smokers. If you are a non-smoker, you may be wondering why people inflict such punishment on themselves.

Have you ever wondered why humans, as smart as we are, tend to be self-destructive?

Are smokers and other addicts really smart? We willfully put poison in our system. Have you even wondered why tobacco companies are allowed to be manufacturing and distributing what essentially is a dangerous killer?

Worldwide, researchers report that there were 1,690,000 premature deaths from cardiovascular disease among smokers in the year 2000. There were approximately 850,000 lung cancer deaths during the same year, and 118,000 COPD deaths from smoking in 2001.

Smoking makes the heart's job difficult, but the fact is, tobacco use plays a role in a multitude of diseases that ultimately lead to disability and or death.

Cigarette smoke is known to contain well over 7,000 chemical compounds; 250 of which are known to be very poisonous and another 70 have been identified as carcinogens.

Many substances have been identified as carcinogenic. Some commonly known carcinogens include asbestos, radon, certain pesticides, arsenic, and tobacco smoke. When viewed in this light, it is no wonder that the effects of smoking are so widespread and destructive.

Smoking Addiction

Smoking addiction is a combination of two types of addiction. There's the physical addiction, then there is the mental, or psychological addiction.

Although nicotine addiction is considered one of the strongest addictions, even more addictive than cocaine, the good news is that the physical side of things doesn't last very long. In fact, some believe that you will lose the physical cravings for nicotine in as little as 7 days.

The real struggle for smokers is overcoming the mental addiction. The smoker has essentially trained their subconscious mind to make smoking an "automatic" behavior.

These are the habits and rituals that a smoker has developed over the years such as smoking when they wake up, just before they go to sleep, after they eat, when they drive, when they drink coffee and/

Or alcohol, and so on.

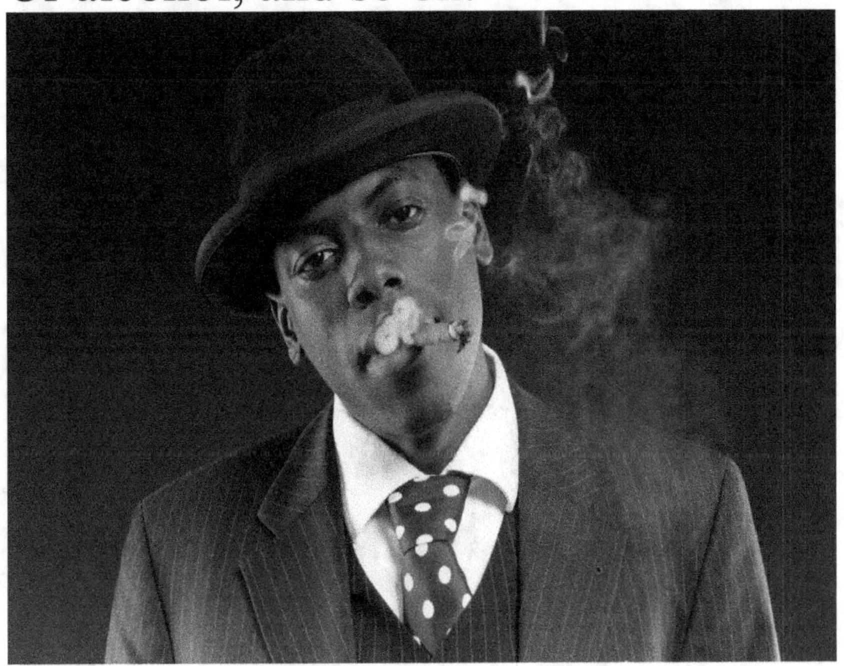

There are many different ways to stub out smoking. Some experts advocate using pharmacological products to help wean you off nicotine while others say all you need is a good counselor and support group.

To add to the confusion, you may find there is a study out there that says this way works better than that one. Then when you research well, you find there is another study that says, no, that one works better than this one.

One thing is true. Most experts agree that a combination of therapies work best.

For instance, nicotine replacement therapy on its own, or counseling on its own is not as effective as a combination of both.

In this book you can read about two of the more common elements of successful easy quit smoking programs.

A lot of Hollywood stars have quit the habit. Stars like Matt Damon, Drew Barrymore, Ben Affleck, Charlize Theron, and Ellen DeGeneres all stubbed out their last cigarettes a long time ago.

They quit smoking using hypnotherapy. Other celebrities have discovered the effective results of hypnotherapy and have used it to conquer their own smoking habits.

Researchers at the University of Iowa combined more than 600 studies of smoking cessation programs involving 72,000 people from North America and Europe.

Hypnosis was found to be over 3 times more effective than nicotine replacement therapy and 15 times more effective than quitting cold turkey.

A comparison study of smoking cessation treatments was conducted by North Shore Medical Center and Massachusetts General Hospital.

26 weeks after discharge, 50% of patients who received hypnotherapy exclusively were non-smokers compared to the 25% of patients who didn't and only 16% of patients who used nicotine replacement therapy alone.

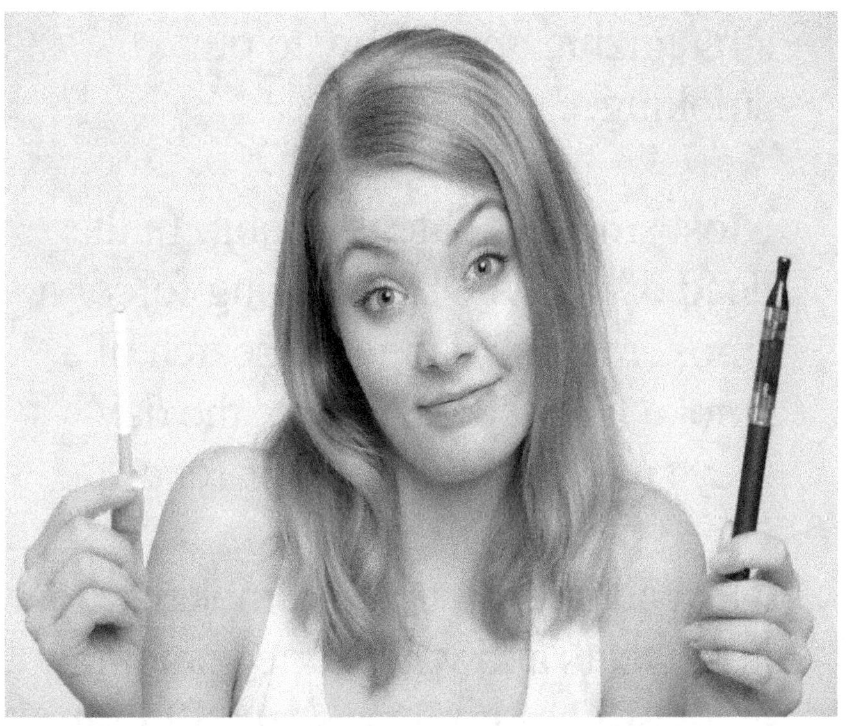

Smokers, usually do not often talk much about it, but we worry about the damage we inflict on ourselves by smoking every hour of everyday.

One more thing we usually do not talk about is how much time we spend every now and then strategizing about how to quit smoking.

Most smokers hate the habit. In the dead of nights when craving forces a smoker to risk danger in search of a smoke, they silently curse the day they smoked their first cigarette.

Most addicts do this. A smoker who is 50 years and who started smoking at age 18 has perhaps spent 30 years thinking of how to quit smoking.

A friend spent 26 of his 36 years as a smoker dreaming wistfully of the day he could call himself an *ex*-smoker and really mean it. Think about it.

That is an awfully long time to continue doing something you really hate, but then, that is the nature of nicotine addiction.

Benefits of Smoking Cessation

- Every breath you take feels clean and refreshing
- You are not quickly tired during the day
- You sleep better at night
- You lose insomnia
- You are a bundle of stamina
- You exude confidence- no worries of smelly mouth
- Your finance improves- Consider $13 * 2 * 365 days
- Sharper thinking
- Pride in self

- Family and friends no longer suffer secondhand smoke
- Confidence in your ability to quit – that is an accomplishment

There are much more

- Your skin is radiant
- Your body starts to repair itself 20 minutes after you quit
- Your gum and teeth recover
- Your heart feels relaxed. It now works with less effort
- Heartburn and indigestion reduces
- You can now appreciate non-smoking restaurants
- No worrying about attending events where you cannot smoke

- Your car smells good
- Your clothing smells better
- Your house smells good
- The chance of setting your house on fire is significantly reduced
- You are now health conscious and you spend accordingly
- No more fear of getting fired for smoking
- No more fear of losing your job because you are reason your company's health insurance premium is high
- You can now get insurance at cheaper premiums
- Your sinus problems are gone
- Allergies and asthma improves
- You have set example for your family and friends
- You can even sing again

- Time wasted smoking is recovered
- Whiter teeth
- If you are single, hey, the chance to meet a friend is greater
- Anxiety level subsides
- No more of those cigarette cough
- Your sense of smell improves
- You appetite get better
- You smell better
- You can breathe

We did not even list the cost of cigarettes that are now savings. This is because the real savings are factored in your quality of life, the illnesses you have avoided and the medical cost both to you, your family and/or the State.

A List of Reasons to Quit

The above is quite enough reasons to quit smoking. If the above reasons are not incentive enough to quit, what you are doing by continuous smoking is akin to buying a gun and threatening to blow your brains out.

The truth of the matter is that you're not threatening. You are already blowing yourself away slowly.

Every cigarette you smoke is one bullet placed in the cylinder and you are pulling the trigger like in Russian roulette.

Give quitting a try. Never mind if you fail. If you fail, try again. Sometimes, it takes 7 tries to a success. This is true in all endeavors. Quitting smoking is no different.

Using medication to help you quit

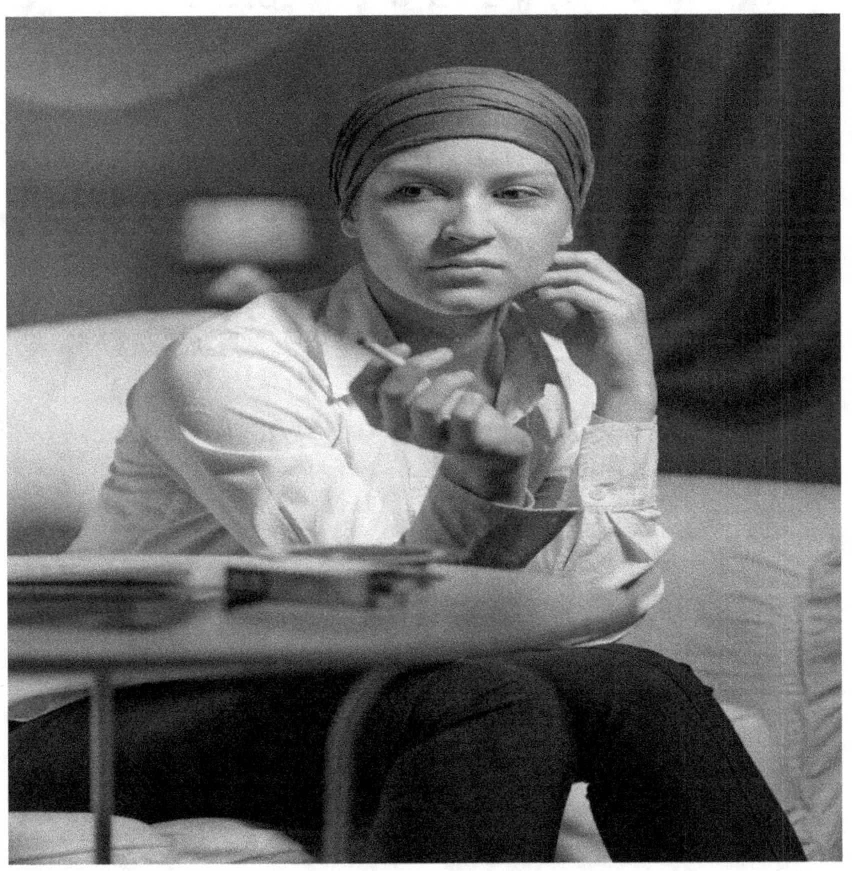

Medicines can help you quit when you use them correctly. Nicotine replacement medicines contain gradually decreasing doses of nicotine to help reduce the headaches and irritability you may have when you quit smoking.

Non-nicotine prescription medicines can also help you quit by making nicotine cravings less severe.

Your doctor or nurse can help you decide if one of these medicines might help you. Your doctor may also decide that using both a nicotine replacement medicine and a non-nicotine replacement medicine may work better for you.

When you talk to your doctor or nurse, ask how to use the medicine. Studies show that many people don't use their quit-smoking medicines correctly. That is a plan and set-up for failure.

If you don't use the medicine properly, it won't work well for you. And there lies the failure.

The last time I took a friend to see my doctor, I can hear the doctor repeating himself many times say the same thing "Yes, you can stop smoking" "You must follow the prescription".

When he turned to me to ask how I was faring with my personal prescriptions, I replied "I QUIT" already.

He was shocked. I quit since January- that was 8 years ago. I empathize with smokers. Some just do not know how to go about quitting.

The information sheet that comes with your medicine tells you exactly how to use the medicine. Follow it. Your longevity of life depends on it.

Your life's longevity is paramount here. Do you want to smoke your life away? Perhaps, you did not answer in the affirmative, however, by continuing to smoke, you are unwittingly smoking away your longevity.

Non-Nicotine Prescriptions

Bupropion hydrochloride is a medicine for depression, but doctors say it also helps people quit smoking. Brand names include

Zyban®, Wellbutrin®, Wellbutrin SR® and Wellbutrin XL® but these medications are also available as generics.

Varenicline is a relatively new medicine that may help smokers quit. It is currently available under the brand name Chantix®. My doctor recommended this and it worked like charm.

You can smoke when you use it. However, the taste of the smoke gradually turns nasty. The number of times you inhale drops. Soon, you cannot even smoke half a stick when you crave smoking.

Soon any attempt to satisfy your cravings turns sour and the craving is forgotten. At this time, your prescription is working. Give it time.

- These prescriptions work by blocking the flow of chemicals in the brain that make you crave and want to smoke.
- Both medicines come in pill form. You start out with a low dose and gradually increase up to the full dose.
- It takes about a week for these medicines to work, so you need to start taking them before you quit smoking.
- Each of these medicines may interact differently with other medicines you are taking.
- Make sure your doctor have a complete list of all your medicines, including over-the-counter drugs.

- You may need to use a non-nicotine prescription medicine for quite a while 3 months or longer- as your doctor recommends.
- When you get ready to stop taking a non-nicotine prescription medicine, you may need to take a gradually decreasing dose before you stop completely.
- The FDA notified the public that the use of varenicline or bupropion has been associated with reports of behavior changes including hostility, agitation, depressed mood, and suicidal thoughts or actions.
- When taking these drugs, if you experience any serious and unusual changes in mood or

behavior or feel like hurting yourself or someone else, you should stop taking the medicine and call your healthcare professional immediately.

- Tell your friends your struggles. Your friends and/or family members who notice unusual changes in your behavior or in someone who is taking varenicline or bupropion for smoking cessation should tell the person their concerns and recommend that you/he or she stop taking the drug and call your doctor immediately.

Hypnotherapy Can Help You Quit

So what will hypnotherapy do? Rather than just treating the physical urges that are part of your smoking habit, hypnotherapy targets the subconscious drive behind the addiction,

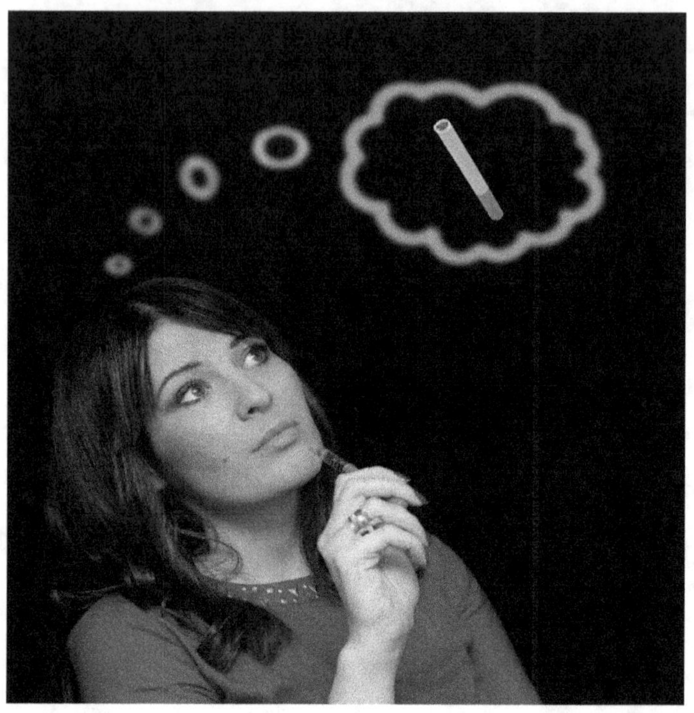

and breaks your positive associations with cigarettes that your mind has formed.

This is replaced by an empowering, smoke-free perspective your hypnotist offers through verbal suggestions that is likely to deem smoking as something undesirable and thus unnecessary.

As the sessions of your hypnotherapy progresses, the suggestions by the hypnotherapist take hold and diminish the smoker's crave for cigarettes.

Furthermore, hypnotherapy is considered to be a far more safe and natural method to quit smoking with and is non-habit forming.

This cannot be said about most of the stop smoking aids we currently have on the market. However, going to a hypnotist can be expensive. As much as $200 per one hour session, and requiring as many as 5 sessions for the entire treatment.

If you're a celebrity like the ones mentioned earlier, then this is not a problem. But can the average smoker afford to go to a hypnotherapist?

Well, that question is left to the individual, but consider that a pack a day smoker will spend in excess of $4000 a year on cigarettes. This does not even include the increased cost on life and health insurance. The cost to a smoker must include the drastic cut in your ability to earn and to live healthy life.

If you live in a location where the government heavily taxes tobacco like New York City, you will be spending for a pack of cigarettes $16 * 365days =$5840.

If you are a 2 packs a day smoker, you are writing approximately $11,680 check to tobacco companies to kill yourself.

Many people in some geographical locations are living on less than $1 a day budget.

Surviving Nicotine Withdrawal

This is it. This the phase that you make or allow to make you. The cravings are intense. All your thoughts are focused. Focused only on the cigarettes.

You need to empower yourself by knowing what to expect and thus prepare yourself accordingly. Follow your doctor's prescriptions to the letter. Nicotine withdrawal is a short phase but it can be very intense.

Things to do when the urge to smoke becomes unbearable:

1. Plan this smoking cessation with your family. You will need their support.
2. Write down the reasons why you want to quit smoking. Carry it on your person.
3. When that urge for just one cigarette becomes unbearable, pull out your list in #2
4. When the thought of smoking begins, take yourself to an incident you think you could have handled differently and seriously think about it.
5. Never rationalize yourself to a cigarette. As soon as you start rationalizing pull out your list in #2 and read it over and over.

6. Reward yourself. For every day you conquered, tell your friends and support persons.
7. Be Patient. It takes time. When the urge to smoke arises, think of immersing yourself in a bathtub full of water and while away the time. You engage in unusual things to conquer each day. Remember nicotine withdrawal lasts a short phase.
8. Play some games, word puzzles etc.
9. Review your reasons for smoking cessation.
10. Change how you think: Instead of you thinking about smoking, think instead the damage cigarettes does to you, your family and friends.

11.   Be ready for weight gains. Be ready for exercise. A few minutes of walk-out. Three times a week will do it.

12.   Watch and pay attention to a handful of TV advertisements on the bad side of smoking cigarettes.

13.   Watch documentaries on the effects of smoking cigarettes. It will boost your resolve. Watch these videos anytime you crave a smoke.

14.   Use your mind. Think the effects of smoking. Remember, your mind is the strongest weapon in this fight.

The game plan above will help you to be more firm about your decision to quit, and will make you committed to the process.

You should pick a date for starting to quit, and check off every day that you have successfully gone without smoking.

 Pick a time of the week or month that will be the most stress-free for you, where you will be less likely to break down and want a cigarette.

This is very important.

You have to remove that macho man's hat. If you were able to control your mind, you would have quit sooner than this.

What are your triggers? Know your triggers. Write down the

triggers that lead you to smoking or smoke more.

Whether it is drinking whisky, going to parties, or even listening to jazz, make plans on how you can avoid your triggers.

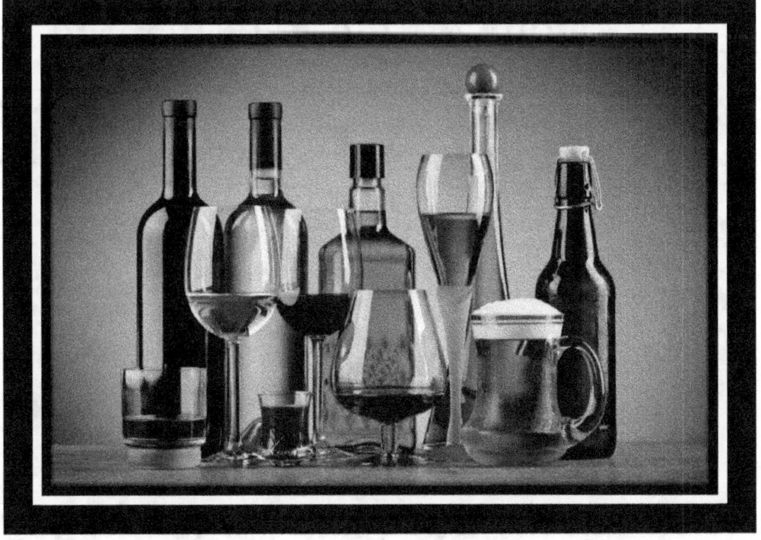

Most smokers say coffee is their worst trigger. Then, avoid coffee in the earlier days. I had a friend tell me that two of his worst triggers were coffee and when he sits in the toilet. He devised a plan to deal with both.

- Keep reminding yourself why you want to quit. Once you start your plan, keep telling yourself that you want to quit for health reasons, for your family, and for your friends. You can even write a motivational note to yourself and keep it in your wallet.
- Remember that the first few days are the hardest. Factor this into your game plan. Give reward to yourself for getting through your first few days, or first few weeks of quitting. It is so important that you do this with your family watching.

- Keep a good journal where you record your thoughts and feelings throughout the process. Make a plan to write in the journal at least once a day so you feel more in touch with how your mind and body are feeling. This is also very important. Do you think you understand how your mind works? Do not toy with your mind.

You just do not understand how it works. Even scientists are at a loss at this moment. And this moment is this day, this month, this year.

You just have to help your mind and its cravings. When it craves something and it don't get it, it starts to adjust its cravings.

Not recommending Quitting Cold Turkey

Perhaps, there are a lot of smokers who have tried to quit by a snap of the finger as if they are under hypnosis.

Of 100 people who try quitting cold turkey, 97 returned to smoking full time. Its failure rate is guaranteed.

It takes courage and determination to stub out that last cigarette and quit smoking. If you think you don't have the courage and determination— think of all the disease and illnesses facing you. You are tempting death.

Most people feel an intense combination of fear, anxiety and excitement leading up to the anticipated quit date.

Feeling afraid to quit smoking is completely normal as it is a by-product of your smoking addiction.

Understand the pros and cons of quitting cold turkey. Quitting cold turkey means deciding to quit smoking completely without the help of nicotine replacement therapy or drugs.

This requires perseverance and independence. Only 3 out of

100 people have been able to successfully quit smoking cold turkey because of the drastic change this makes in their lives.

Before you try quitting cold turkey, you should understand the advantages and disadvantages of the process. I do not recommend quitting cold turkey unless you suddenly are diagnosed with life threatening illness.

Quitting cold turkey will guarantee you to experience intense and unpleasant withdrawal symptoms, such as depression, insomnia, irritability, and anxiety. On top of all that, you have less of a chance of success if you quit cold turkey than if you try to use a combination of other methods listed above.

For most addictions in life, there are minimal successes when the attempt to quit is done cold turkey.

Babies teach us that very well. They have to learn over a period of time to sit, crawl and finally take a few wobbly steps.

Over time they walk well and steady and finally they run. They learned.

Smokers are like babies. You have to learn to reduce the number of cigarettes smoked in one day.

If you smoke 2 packets a day, you did not start smoking 2 packs from the first day you smoked.

It was a build up to a packet then 2 packets. So learn to turn that build up to build down.

Choose the time frame you think you can slowly reduce your cigarette consumption from two pack a day to one pack a day.

The Program

Here it comes:

Let us say we chose one year time frame to quit. Work with me here:

One year---------12 months.

@ 2 packs a day ---------40 cigarettes

Month 1 subtract 6 sticks from 40 = you smoke 34 sticks a day

Month 2 subtract 10 sticks from 40   = you smoke 30 sticks a day

Month 3 subtract 15 sticks
from 40   =you
smoke 25

Month 4 subtract 20 sticks
from 40   = you smoke 1
packet. Give yourself some
treats- You are half way there.
You are building down
gradually. And you are loving
the feeling. Congratulations!

Month 5 minus 5 from 1packet
= you smoke 15

Month 6 minus 8 from 1packet
= you make do with 12 sticks

Month 7 subtract 10 from
1packet   = you smoke
10 sticks. Way-To- Go.

Month 8 subtract 12 from
1packet   = you smoke 8
sticks a day

Month 9 subtract 14 from
1packet   = 6 sticks
(Now, you smoking less than a
packet in 3 days).

Kudos! WAY TO GO!

You have added days and weeks to your life span and longevity. You are about to cut off some of the illnesses smokers are likely to suffer from.

At this rate, you have reclaimed about 2 months to your longevity. The 2 months that would otherwise been lost to cigarette.

If you smoked 4 packets, you reclaimed 4 months.

At this rate (6 sticks a day) you are still, however, losing days of your life to smoking.

So, keep at it.

Month 10 subtract 16 from 1packet   = you have only 4 sticks a day- Do not cheat- Your mind's eye is watching you.

Ask your family to watch and help you too. Tell your friends that you smoke 4 sticks a day only.

If you have come this far, you are a genius. You are

determined and nothing must stop you now. Kudos!

Can you imagine that now you are smoking one packet in 5days?

Yes you can do it. You are almost there.

Month 11- You are now on ONLY TWO STICKS a day – one after breakfast and one before going to bed. You may want to save the one for the morning for later.

You can push it to noon. Get ready to see your doctor. Some smokers are likely to see their doctor at this stage or before. You don't have a doctor? Check out programs run by

City on quitting smoking. You will get help there.

Your chance of kicking the habit now with a prescription of Chantix is very high. Your chance of success is equal or greater than 90 percent.

YOUR LAST MONTH:

Still on 2 sticks. Make the doctor's appointment. Get your pills (Chantix).

Follow the prescription religiously. Keep smoking the 2 sticks as you administer your Chantix. Don't worry because with the medications, the urge to smoke subsides until you start yelling "Damn! I did not smoke yesterday…last week…last month."

You have won.

You have conquered the demon urging you to crave and smoke.

Soon, you will begin to notice other smokers as you begin to feel empathize with them.

If you smoked 100 sticks a day- that is 5 packs a day. You lucky to be still alive. To start on the above program, subtract 66 sticks to qualify to follow the program.

4 packets a day------------ subtract 46 sticks on Month 1

3 packets a day-----------
subtract 26 sticks on Month 1

GOOD LUCK!

When this approach works for you, do not forget your friends and colleagues who are also smokers.

You just set an example. Please share your success and encourage them to quit.

Give this e-book as a gift. Let us quit smoking cigarettes. Yes you can smoke to quit.

Other Kindle books by this author are listed below.

1.

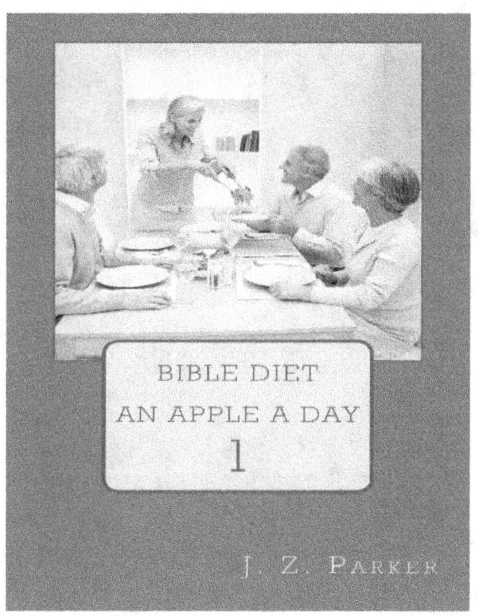

Gen 1:29 Then God said, "I give you every seed-bearing plant on the face of the whole earth and every tree that has fruit with seed in it. They will be yours for food. Gen 1:30 And to all the beasts of the earth and all the birds in the sky and all the creatures that move along the ground--everything that has the

breath of life in it--I give every green plant for food." And it was so.

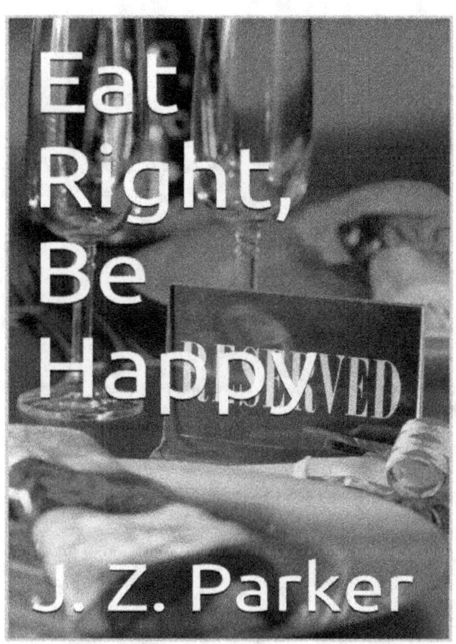

2.

Most often, being overweight is as a result of incapacitation. Overweight is a direct result of damaged communication between the body and the brain.

To some overweight individuals, the reward is in the food at all times from beginning to when the last piece of the food is eaten. Any more food brought immediately will still have the same reward.

3. Empower Your DNA: The Power of Vitamin C.

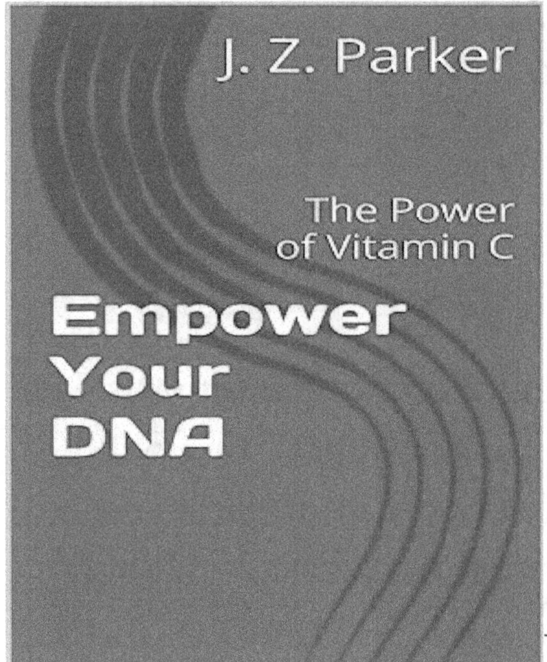

Many scientifically controlled studies using vitamin C for colds show that it can reduce the severity of cold symptoms, acting as a natural antihistamine. It can also be very useful for allergy control for the same reason: It reduces histamine levels. Because vitamin C gives your immune system one of the important nutrients it needs, extra vitamin C would often shorten the duration of the cold as well.

Banana Blossoms: Banana Flowers:

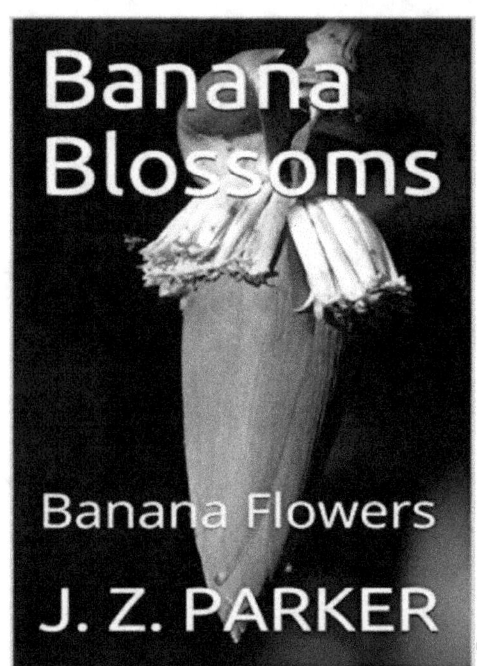

The most ignored and perhaps never eaten part of a banana tree, can reverse aging, diabetes and polycystic ovary syndrome (PCOS). There are so many other health benefits, so much so, you may wonder why we have not known about this part of a banana tree sooner.

It has been a staple in most Asian countries. It can be prepared in many different ways in soups, stews, salads and sandwiches. This is one vegetable you need to eat regularly. It is worth it.

Good & Bad Plastics: Bisphenol A:

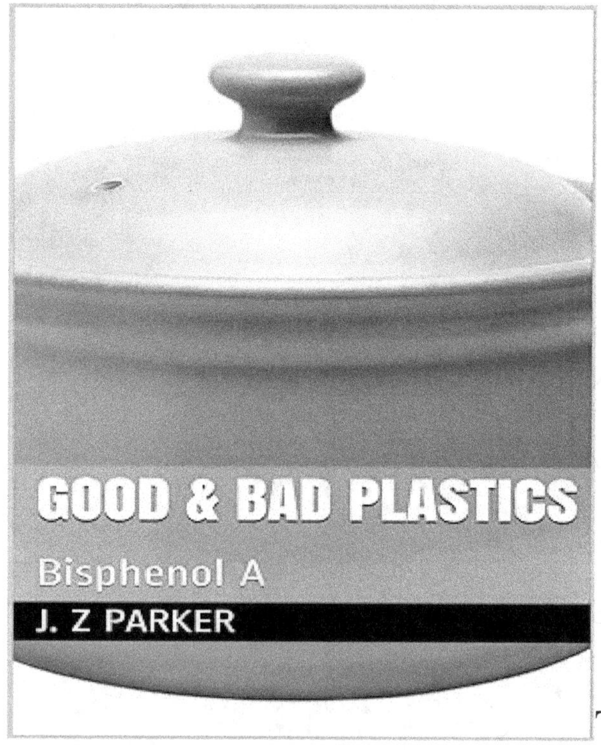

The wonder of canned food. Whip it open, heat it up in a plastic container and voilà, your meal is served. What is wrong with this picture? Did you notice the double whammy there? Some canned foods can affect your sex life negatively. They can also affect your libido negatively. How is your food stored? If you buy canned foods—any can—then read on.